MENOPAUSE NATURALLY

A Holistic Guide to a Smooth Transition

by Kathleen Fry, M.D., and
Claudia Wingo, R.N., Medical Herbalist

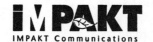
IMPAKT Communications

Health Information Specialists

www.impakt.com

Published by:
IMPAKT Communications, Inc.
P.O. Box 12496
Green Bay, WI 54307-2496
Phone: (920) 434-3838
Fax: (920) 434-8884
E-mail: info@impakt.com
www.impakt.com

Dedication

This book is dedicated to the many healthcare professionals who have been true trailblazers in the area of women's health. Most of all, this book is dedicated to the thousands of patients we have treated over the years and the countless more we hope to touch with our information.

Acknowledgements

Many people played a significant role in creating this book. First and foremost, we would like to thank IMPAKT Communications Publisher Karolyn A. Gazella, IMPAKT Editor Frances E. FitzGerald, and Assistant Editor Holly Hurst. We also thank the book's designer, Tami Schommer, and the entire IMPAKT staff.

Our special thanks go to Dr. Haru Amagase, Brenda Petesch, and the staff of Wakunaga of America, manufacturers and distributors of Estro•Logic®, the menopause formula we designed. Thanks also to our Canadian product distributor, Quest Vitamins.

We are enormously grateful to our families and friends. They have supported us during our professional search for quality information and innovative ways to satisfy the needs of our patients.

Foreword
by Karolyn A. Gazella
president and founder,
IMPAKT Communications, Inc.,
author of *Buyer Be Wise*,
co-author of *Activate Your Immune System*

At the age of 33, I was diagnosed with ovarian cancer. The complete hysterectomy caused surgically induced menopause. While my cancer prognosis looked good, my doctor prescribed hormone replacement therapy for my menopausal symptoms. My strong family history of breast cancer caused me to question this decision. I was told that there were no other options, and that if I wanted symptom relief I had to take the prescription.

As a research journalist and health writer, I naturally began to investigate other options. I was also too stubborn to simply "grin and bear" my symptoms of menopause, which at times could become drastic. It seemed I had it all: hot flashes, night sweats, depression, mood changes, and vaginal dryness. At times, I thought the menopause was more challenging than the cancer!

I have been involved in the natural health industry for more than 10 years. I realized very quickly that my solutions were right in front of me. Within months of my surgery, I began using a more natural approach to alleviate my menopausal symptoms. Within weeks, my natural approach began working.

Today, five years later, I can happily report that I am not only cancer-free, but I am also free of menopausal symptoms. Similar to the recommendations of Dr. Fry and Claudia Wingo, I utilize a comprehensive plan that includes dietary changes, increased exercise, nutritional supplements, and mind/body techniques.

I am proud to be associated with this book by Dr. Fry and Ms. Wingo. It represents an effective program for women who are seeking alternatives to conventional drug therapy. I am confident this book will help many women reach the success I have achieved.

Contents

"The most creative force in the world
is the post-menopausal woman with zest."
—Margaret Mead

Introduction

The need to know, the right to choose

The female body is a complex blend of physical and emotional components, all trying to achieve the same goal—balance. The female reproductive system is controlled by a sophisticated, internal team of hormones that influence nearly every aspect of our lives. Hormones influence how we look, feel, think, and act. When hormones are doing their job, they promote internal harmony. When hormones are not in balance, chaos can result.

Menopause is characterized by hormonal imbalance. As healthcare professionals, we have seen patients who breeze through menopause without any problems. We've also seen patients who are nearly incapacitated by their symptoms. Menopause is unique for every woman.

"Menopause, when understood and supported, provides the next level of initiation into personal power for women," writes author Tamara Slayton in her book, *Reclaiming the Menstrual Matrix*. Christiane Northrup, M.D., author of *Women's Bodies Women's Wisdom*, calls the years following menopause "the wisdom years."

Menopause can represent a new, positive beginning in a woman's life. However, the woman who experiences uncomfortable and sometimes debilitating menopausal symptoms may not perceive this as a vibrant time of her life, filled with limitless opportunities. This woman is not thinking of the great potential that awaits her; instead, she is seeking fast and effective symptom relief. It is for these women that we have written this book. The countless women who are approaching this life-changing stage must be aware that they don't need to suffer.

The natural program outlined in this book will help ease this important transition, allowing women to get on with the business at hand—living life with peace, joy, and vitality.

Female baby-boomers are now reaching this important half-way point in their lives. It has been estimated that by the year 2020, more than 60 million women in North America will be experiencing menopause. That's a lot of women searching for answers to their individual menopause dilemma. As healthcare professionals, we want to inform as many of these women as possible that they do have choices. Armed with the proper knowledge, a woman can truly take advantage of "the wisdom years."

A message from Dr. Fry

In my clinical practice, my focus is helping women experience a smooth menopausal transition. In fact, more than 50 of my patients are enrolled in an open-label clinical study to help determine the effectiveness of an all-natural nutritional supplement for menopause. As a medical doctor, I rely on scientific substantiation, as well as input from my patients. This clinical trial, which will last six months, will give me both.

Over the years, I have witnessed the many side effects associated with conventional hormone replacement therapy. One of the big problems that presently exists is the over-medication of women with mild symptoms, who are just beginning to go through menopause. It's not just the excessive prescribing of estrogens (i.e., Premarin®) and progestins (i.e., Provera®), but also of antidepressants.

Here is a typical scenario: A woman may experience some emotional symptoms, such as forgetfulness or irritability. She visits her family doctor and gets a prescription for antidepressant medication. This is a common occurrence because the early symptoms of menopause often resemble symptoms of depression. However, the hormonal fluctuations typical of this perimenopausal period are not addressed; therefore, the patient does not experience relief from her symptoms or a return to her previous sense of well-being.

Many of my patients have reported a variety of side effects from conventional prescription estrogen and/or progestin. In addition to weight gain and breast tenderness, several of these women say, "I feel bloated and fat" while on the medication. Some indicate that they feel "toxic" or over-medicated when they take certain prescription hormones, such as conjugated equine estrogens.

If you are one of these women, or are considering a conventional prescription for your menopausal symptoms, recognize that you do have options.

Nurse and medical herbalist Claudia Wingo and I will outline a popular option that I presently use in my clinical practice. I am happy to report that patients who have chosen this option are experiencing symptom relief without side effects. You can, too!

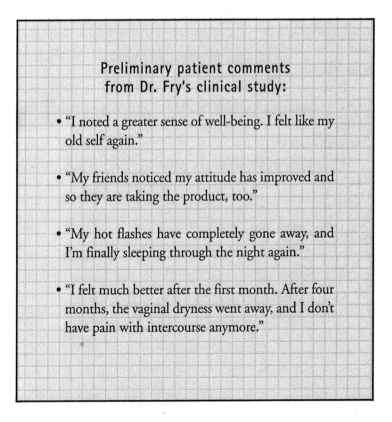

Preliminary patient comments from Dr. Fry's clinical study:

- "I noted a greater sense of well-being. I felt like my old self again."

- "My friends noticed my attitude has improved and so they are taking the product, too."

- "My hot flashes have completely gone away, and I'm finally sleeping through the night again."

- "I felt much better after the first month. After four months, the vaginal dryness went away, and I don't have pain with intercourse anymore."

A message from Claudia Wingo

After my formalized schooling, I became interested in herbal and nutritional medicine. Today, a large percentage of my clients are women. About 65 percent of my menopausal patients experience hot flashes or night sweats that are becoming severe. The other 35 percent experience psychological problems such as memory loss, brain fog, poor concentration, and depression. One patient said she felt as if her "brain had turned into molasses."

To treat this patient population, a comprehensive approach is necessary. Menopause is an especially significant opportunity for a woman to re-evaluate her life. She should specifically look at her diet, exercise habits, and stress levels.

In our culture, women seem to have a more difficult time making a smooth transition. This is different for Asian women. Epidemiological data indicate that fewer than 25 percent of menopausal Japanese women complain of hot flashes, compared with 85 percent of North American women. This is thought to be primarily due to the high consumption of soy foods in Japan.

Because the typical American diet is very low in plant-based foods, women are not getting the natural phytoestrogens they need to help balance hormones. Soy, vegetables, and legumes are just a few great foods that can help ease menopausal symptoms.

Women should focus on taking control of their health through diet, exercise, and nutritional supplements. As a medical herbalist, I have found that herbs provide relief without the side effects of conventionally prescribed estrogen. It is rewarding to see my patients get results and relief.

In 1999, I had the pleasure of meeting Dr. Kathleen Fry at a botanical workshop I was teaching. We began a collaboration that has resulted in a unique supplement that includes a combination of herbal extracts. We are proud to share our information in this book.

Chapter One

Mechanics of menopause

While we don't want to bore you with a lot of technical details about the function of the female reproductive system, we do want to provide some general information. We learned in Biology 101 that, on average, a young female will menstruate every 28 days. What you may not know is that when an infant girl is born, she has the most eggs in her ovaries than she will ever have.

During childhood, the ovaries basically lie dormant and the endometrium (i.e., lining of the uterus) is inactive. The brain is really the first organ involved in hormone regulation. The hypothalamus and anterior pituitary begin to control all the hormonal systems. The pituitary produces follicle-stimulating hormone (FSH) and luteinizing hormone (LH). This is important because these two hormones regulate the ovaries' production of estrogen.

Here's how they work: At puberty, the hypothalamus begins to raise levels of FSH and LH. The result is the menstrual cycle. The rise of FSH every month stimulates the eggs to grow in the ovaries. This process produces estrogen, which stimulates the thickening of the uterine lining to prepare for the embryo. When LH peaks, it stimulates the follicle to rupture, which releases the egg from the ovary. This is, of course, known as ovulation. The egg then makes its way down the fallopian tubes to be fertilized by sperm.

The hormone progesterone stimulates changes in the uterine lining (endometrium) to nourish the developing embryo. Once progesterone is produced, estrogen levels drop. After progesterone is no longer produced, the endometrium sloughs off and menses

28-DAY MENSTRUAL CYCLE SUMMARY

Days 1-5	Days 6-14	Day 14	Days 14-28
• Decline of estrogen and progesterone hormones signals uterus that pregnancy has not occurred. • Bleeding begins. • Follicle-stimulating hormone (FSH) rises, causing follicles in the ovaries to grow, prior to ovulation.	• Estrogen rises. • FSH begins to fall. • Endometrial lining of the uterus thickens, in preparation for possible implantation of the fertilized egg.	• Estrogen helps stimulate large and sudden release of luteinizing hormone (LH), a hormone secreted to cause ovulation. • LH surge causes follicle to rupture, and the egg is expelled into the fallopian tube.	• Immediately after ovulation, the follicle bursts and becomes a corpus luteum. • The corpus luteum begins secreting large amounts of progesterone. • If the egg is not fertilized, the corpus luteum continues to release progesterone for only 14 days. • The process begins again.

(i.e., menstrual period) occurs. When everything runs smoothly, this is an approximately 28-day cycle for the average woman.

In addition to controlling the reproductive process, hormones also regulate neurotransmitters and endorphins (i.e., "feel-good" chemicals) in the brain. Anyone who has experienced premenstrual syndrome (PMS) knows that if her hormones are out of balance, she will have more intense feelings around the time of her menses.

Estrogen, progesterone, FSH, and LH must perform their designated duties throughout a woman's menstruating life in order to maintain hormonal balance.

Perimenopause

The years just prior to menopause are known as perimenopause. This is a time when a woman is still menstruating but may experience some symptoms of menopause. During this time, estrogen and progesterone levels begin to decline. In an effort to compensate for this decline, the pituitary stimulates the ovaries to make more estrogen by releasing more FSH. However, because women have fewer follicles as they age, they cannot produce the needed estrogen. Therefore, there is not enough estrogen to stimulate the LH surge. Without LH, there is no progesterone. And without progesterone, there is no menstruation. Women begin to skip cycles and experience other symptoms of menopause/perimenopause.

Perimenopausal symptoms can include:
- Anxiety and/or depression;
- Formication (a feeling of "ants crawling under the skin");
- Heart palpitations;
- Hot flashes and/or night sweats;
- Inflammation of the vagina;
- Insomnia and/or irritability;
- Muscle and joint aches;
- Poor concentration and/or poor memory;
- Tiredness/fatigue;
- Reduced libido;
- Urinary incontinence; and
- Vaginal dryness and/or vaginal or urinary tract infections.

During the perimenopausal phase, these symptoms last for about a year in 80 percent of women, and for up to five years in 20 percent of women. Perimenopause is typically diagnosed when a woman is over 40 and experiencing erratic periods and other menopausal symptoms.

Transition to menopause is an ongoing process that can vary in length. Most women do not experience an immediate menopause unless surgery is involved. This is also referred to as surgically induced menopause, which occurs when the ovaries are removed prior to perimenopause or menopause. Because surgically induced menopause is not a gradual process, the symptoms may be more frequent and more pronounced. Fortunately, the program outlined in this book can also help women with surgically induced menopause, if their symptoms are mild or moderate. Women with more severe symptoms usually require hormone replacement. However, a compounding pharmacist can individually tailor an alternative to synthetic hormones in the form of bio-identical estrogen and progesterone.

Menopause

Menopause occurs "officially" two years after a woman stops menstruating. By the age of 55, 95 percent of women reach menopause. It typically occurs between the ages of 45 and 60.

At menopause, the ovaries stop producing eggs and estrogen, and progesterone levels decline dramatically. Keep in mind, however, that the ovaries are not the only sources of estrogen in the body. While the ovaries are the biggest producer of estrogen, it is also made in much smaller amounts in the adrenal glands, liver, kidneys, and even in body fat. That's why women who are a little heavier often report fewer menopausal symptoms.

Menopause has been described as a transformation from reproductive to non-reproductive stages. This description is troubling because it sounds as if the woman herself is no longer productive. Drug companies' advertising campaigns often promote a negative attitude about menopause. Many women are brainwashed to believe that to be "forever young" and vibrant, they need estrogen, usually in the form of conjugated estrogens from pregnant mare's urine.

The fact is, the post-menopausal years can be a personal renaissance. If managed properly, menopause can be a time of renewal and revitalization—an end to physical fertility, but a rebirth of the female spirit.

Chapter Two

Choosing conventional treatment

While we advocate our natural menopause program as a treatment plan of first choice, you should be informed about all your options. Most conventional medical doctors utilize prescription drugs as treatments of first choice.

When a woman tells her doctor about symptoms associated with hormonal imbalance, one of two scenarios typically occurs:

1. She is mis-diagnosed and given antidepressants, or

2. She is given an estrogen drug.

As women learn more about the drawbacks of estrogen drugs, more of them are searching for natural alternatives. That wasn't always the case, however.

The most commonly prescribed estrogen drug is known as Premarin®. Since its introduction in the 1970s, Premarin has been one of the most frequently prescribed drugs in the United States. In 1996, more than 22 million prescriptions for Premarin were written in the United States alone. It is one of the top 10 drugs prescribed in the United States today.

"The routine prescription of Premarin fails to take women's individual needs, background, and lifestyles into account," explains Marla Ahlgrimm, R.Ph., founder of Women's Health America, PMS Access, and Madison Pharmacy, the nation's first pharmacy specializing in women's health and natural hormone replacement therapy. "The idea that an off-the-shelf recipe can be appropriate for all women is not only incorrect, but in many cases, this standardized approach actually harms women's health and well-being."

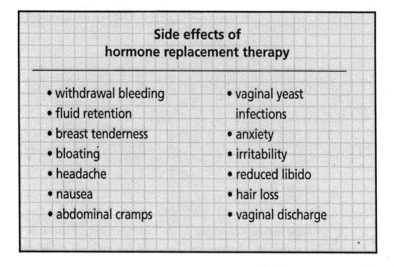

Side effects of hormone replacement therapy

- withdrawal bleeding
- fluid retention
- breast tenderness
- bloating
- headache
- nausea
- abdominal cramps
- vaginal yeast infections
- anxiety
- irritability
- reduced libido
- hair loss
- vaginal discharge

According to the *Physician's Desk Reference®* (*PDR*), several side effects are associated with Premarin, including withdrawal bleeding, fluid retention, breast tenderness, bloating, headache, nausea, abdominal cramps, vaginal yeast infections, anxiety, irritability, reduced libido, hair loss, and vaginal discharge. It is ironic, and incredibly unfortunate, that many menopausal symptoms are, in fact, the very side effects of the medication doctors are prescribing for those symptoms.

Furthermore, these types of prescription estrogens, known clinically as conjugated estrogens, have been shown to increase a woman's risk of developing uterine and breast cancer. Author Susan M. Lark, M.D., clarified the estrogen/breast cancer controversy in her book, *The Estrogen Decision.* The Nurses' Health study, published in the June 1995 *New England Journal of Medicine,* reported that women who took prescription estrogen for five or more years had a 30 to 40 percent higher incidence of breast cancer than those who were not on hormone replacement therapy.

In addition to uterine and breast cancer, hormone replacement therapy (HRT) can cause blood-clotting problems, high blood pressure, and gallbladder disease. HRT is not recommended for women who have gallbladder disease or abnormal menstrual bleeding.

The Premarin approach is not only riddled with side effects and risks, it is like trying to make all women wear a size 2 pair of slacks—for the majority of women, it just doesn't fit!

Occasionally, the natural program outlined in this book does not provide the relief a patient is looking for. For these difficult-to-treat cases, we usually prescribe a combination of estriol and estradiol. An estriol/estradiol prescription must be obtained from a physician and is made by a compounding pharmacist. The pharmacist can make it in either a cream or pill form. For women with severe symptoms, we also often prescribe progesterone cream. In addition to relieving symptoms and promoting overall hormonal balance, progesterone helps prevent osteoporosis.

In addition to the promise of symptom relief, many women take prescribed estrogen because they are told it will decrease their risk of two life-threatening illnesses: heart disease and osteoporosis. Let's take a closer look at each of these serious health conditions.

Heart disease

Scientific studies have confirmed that estrogen increases "good" cholesterol (i.e., HDL) and decreases "bad" cholesterol (i.e., LDL). For this reason, it is assumed that estrogen can reduce the risk of developing heart disease. However, estrogen therapy increases the risk of blood clotting and high blood pressure. Seems contradictory, doesn't it?

It is true that many studies have shown that estrogen benefits the heart. However, our comprehensive plan utilizes other heart-healthy techniques, such as diet, lifestyle factors, and nutritional supplements. Here are some of our key heart-healthy recommendations:

- **Diet.** Increase consumption of pure water, fiber, and fresh vegetables, while decreasing your intake of high-fat foods, refined sugar, alcohol, and caffeine.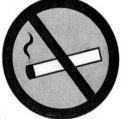
- **Lifestyle factors.** Increase physical activity, decrease stress, and if you smoke, QUIT!
- **Nutritional supplements.** Supplement your diet with a comprehensive multivitamin/mineral formula. Also take aged garlic extract, which reduces multiple cardiovascular disease factors and may reduce breast cancer risk.
- **Regular aerobic exercise**, preferably outdoors in clean air, is beneficial.
- **Stress reduction techniques**, such as yoga and meditation, can help protect the heart.

There are many natural ways to reduce your risk of heart disease. Before turning to estrogen therapy, you may want to consider a more natural heart-healthy program.

NOTE: If you are experiencing symptoms of heart disease or have a strong family history of heart disease, be sure to consult your physician. Never discontinue any medication without first talking to your doctor. Self-diagnosis and self-treatment can be dangerous and are not recommended.

Osteoporosis

Osteoporosis is characterized by a decrease in bone mineral density and a deterioration of bone structure. Osteoporotic bones are porous and fracture easily. Bone mineral density is determined by a complex interplay of minerals, of which calcium is the primary component.

You may think bone tissue is hard, lifeless material. Bone is actually made up of living tissue that is constantly changing and regenerating itself. In fact, every eight years, we have a whole new skeleton.

Unfortunately, increased consumption of nutrient-depleted foods and items (such as caffeine, alcohol, and tobacco) sap calcium from our bones. That and a variety of other factors have triggered an increase in the incidence of osteoporosis. It has been called a "silent epidemic," because it can exist without any symptoms until a fracture occurs.

The National Osteoporosis Foundation has reported that one in two women over the age of 50 is likely to experience an osteoporosis-related fracture in her lifetime. Nearly 30 million Americans, 80 percent of whom are women, have either osteoporosis or low bone density. The National Osteoporosis Foundation predicts that, if left unchecked, 41 million people will be diagnosed with osteoporosis or low bone density by the year 2015. Osteoporosis has become a major public health concern.

While estrogen therapy has been shown to benefit bone strength, we question whether the benefit is worth the side effects. As clinicians, we are always asking ourselves, "is there a better way?" The fact is, weak bones are a result of more than simply a decline in estrogen. Most women don't realize that about 50 percent of bone loss occurs before menopause even begins.

"Statistics show that six to 18 percent of women between 25 and 35 years of age have abnormally low bone density," according to women's wellness expert Christiane Northrup, M.D.

In our search for "a better way" to prevent and treat osteoporosis, we have focused on nutrients such as calcium, magnesium, vitamin D, boron, vitamin K, and other trace minerals, such as strontium and vanadium.

• Adequate **calcium** intake is essential for optimum bone health. We recommend 1,000mg per day, based upon the RDI (recommended daily intake). No more than 400mg of calcium can be absorbed at any one time, so if you take calcium only in supplemental form, take it in divided dosages. Good food sources of calcium include:

— Yogurt (8 oz or one cup plain) = 452mg
— Skim or 1 to 2 percent milk (8 oz or one cup) = 375mg
— Almonds (1 cup) = 355mg
— Tofu (1/2 cup firm) = 260mg
— Cheddar cheese (1 oz) or salmon (canned 3 oz) = 200mg
— Cottage cheese (8 oz) = 160mg
— Mozzarella cheese (1 oz) = 150mg
— Broccoli (1/2 cup cooked) = 90mg

• **Vitamin D** has been shown to promote calcium absorption. The recommended dietary allowance (RDA) for vitamin D is 400 IU. Vitamin D is a fat-soluble vitamin and more than 800 IU is not recommended. Good dietary sources of vitamin D are cold-water fish such as mackerel, salmon, and herring.

• **Vitamin C** may work with calcium to enhance bone development, suggests recent research.

• **Magnesium** is also an important mineral. Some experts believe it is just as important as calcium for bone health. Nearly 60 percent of the magnesium in the human body is concentrated in the bones. According to Dr. Northrup, "A diet low in magnesium and relatively high in calcium can actually contribute to osteoporosis." Too much calcium can deplete the body's stores of magnesium. Most natural health experts recommend magnesium-to-calcium in a 1:2 ratio (e.g., 500mg of magnesium for every 1,000mg of calcium). Good food sources of magnesium include tofu, legumes, seeds, nuts, whole grains, and green vegetables.

The next chapter will discuss why soy is a great food for women experiencing menopausal symptoms. Not only does soy help alleviate symptoms, it also benefits the heart and strengthens bones. Soy is a great source of dietary calcium as well as other bone-building and heart-healthy nutrients.

Osteoporosis
Risk Factors

- POOR DIET

- SMOKING

- CAFFEINE

- CARBONATED
  SOFT DRINKS

- ALCOHOL

- SEDENTARY
  LIFESTYLE

- AGE AND
  GENDER

- FAMILY
  HISTORY

- BODY WEIGHT

- HORMONE
  STATUS

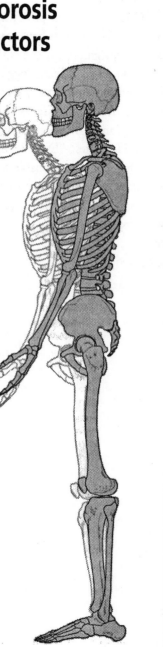

Get moving!

One of the most powerful osteoporosis treatments known is exercise. Many studies have confirmed that a lack of regular physical activity significantly contributes to osteoporosis. Weight-bearing exercises such as walking, jogging, and aerobics help maintain bone mass and protect against osteoporosis.

Dr. Freedolph Anderson writes in his book, *Build Bone Health*, that yoga and light weight training help prevent osteoporosis of the spine. He states, "Exercise is perhaps the most powerful medicine available to us today. It can help enhance self-image, alleviate depression and anxiety, and help prevent chronic, degenerative diseases like osteoporosis."

Chapter Three

Finding relief through diet and lifestyle

Here is some great news for women struggling with menopause: The diet you follow to alleviate symptoms of menopause will also protect against serious illnesses such as cancer and heart disease. When you add healthy lifestyle choices, you dramatically increase your likelihood of achieving optimal health and longevity.

We can tell you from our direct, clinical experience that diet and lifestyle factors are the two most critical components of a successful natural menopause treatment program. Our many patients are living proof that this comprehensive program works. The first step is realizing that you have the power to change your situation. What you do every day will either improve or worsen your symptoms.

Let's start with diet. Here is our seven-point plan for successful menopause symptom control:

1. **Eat organic whenever possible.** Organic foods allow you to avoid harmful preservatives, additives, pesticides, and most importantly, hormones. Replace artificial sweeteners, such as aspartame, with natural sweeteners, such as honey, molasses, and the herb, stevia. Add more fresh, whole, unprocessed foods to your diet.

2. Reduce or eliminate your consumption of red meat. Red meat tends to be higher in saturated fat and lower in nutrient content. Furthermore, growth hormones are often given to animals to increase their size. When we eat meat, we ingest these hormones, which may contribute to the growth of cancer cells. Also, too much protein in the diet can interfere with calcium metabolism and contribute to osteoporosis.

3. Eat more plant foods. Vegetables, grains, fruits, seeds, and nuts are great sources of important phytoestrogens. These will help relieve your menopausal symptoms and contribute to overall health (we'll discuss phytoestrogens in more detail in the next chapter).

4. Avoid fried foods and convenience/ "junk" foods. These foods provide little nutrition and can make menopausal symptoms worse. Fried foods can also weaken the immune system and damage the heart. It is always best to steam, bake, broil, or poach.

5. Reduce or eliminate your intake of caffeine, refined sugar, and salt. These substances can make symptoms worse and are not good choices for overall health. Many women report that caffeine, in particular, makes hot flashes flare. Caffeine also acts as a diuretic, which may contribute to calcium loss.

6. Reduce or eliminate your intake of alcohol and carbonated soft drinks. Alcohol has been linked to an increased risk of developing breast cancer. It can also exacerbate menopausal symptoms, especially hot flashes and insomnia. Soft drinks have been shown to deplete calcium and other minerals from bones.

7. **Eat more soy, tofu, miso, and soybeans.** Soy is such an important food that we need to explore it further.

More soy, please

The scientific community is recognizing the incredible health benefits of soy. Soy foods have been shown to help:

- alleviate menopausal symptoms such as hot flashes and night sweats;
- lower cholesterol and benefit heart health;
- increase bone mineral density to prevent osteoporosis; and
- stimulate immune defenses against certain cancers.

That's a powerful food! Soybeans contain high amounts of protein, calcium, magnesium, iron, zinc, B-vitamins, vitamin E, and essential fatty acids. In addition, soy contains unique health-promoting compounds known as isoflavones. These isoflavones have been studied extensively throughout the world.

The scientific research on soy and the heart is so strong that in 1999, the United States Food and Drug Administration (FDA) allowed food products containing soy protein to carry a label promoting soy's benefits for heart health. The FDA made this endorsement based on compelling evidence that soy helps reduce "bad" (LDL) cholesterol, while preserving "good" (HDL) cholesterol.

According to registered dietitian Patti Tveit Milligan, M.S., R.D., "The soybean may be small in size, but science is confirming that it packs a huge punch when it comes to protecting and enhancing your health."

Recipes with beneficial foods

Because diet is such a critical part of the smooth transition program, we've included a few of our favorite recipes. Enjoy!

SAVORY POTATO AND LEEK SOUP

You can serve this soup steaming hot in the winter or well chilled in the summer. It's a treat either way.

    1 Tbsp. butter
    1 white onion, chopped
    3-4 cloves garlic
    3 medium leeks, *very* well washed and chopped
        (make sure you split them and wash well between
        the leaves; nothing is worse than grit in your soup)

Sauté the above ingredients in a crockpot, then add:
    3 medium/large potatoes, peeled and chopped
    1 pkg. soft tofu, blended till smooth in food processor
    1 tsp. celery salt
    1/2 tsp. ground pepper
    1 tsp. thyme, dried, or 2 tsp. fresh
    1/2 tsp. marjoram, dried, or 1 tsp. fresh
    1 Tbsp. chives, dried, or 2 Tbsp. fresh
    Enough water to fill crockpot 7/8 full

Turn on low for 3-6 hours. You can serve this soup chunky if desired but it is traditionally pureed in the blender or food processor. For a really decadent creamy soup, stir in 1 cup cream, or you can use a soy cream for extra isoflavones. Serve hot, or chill for several hours for a summer soup. Top with chopped chive and thyme.

THAI CHICKPEA SOUP

This soup is a real blend of cultures: Turkish, Italian, and Thai. This is the one time I soak the peas overnight, as chickpeas take longer to cook than any others.

    1 red onion, chopped
    1 red bell pepper, sliced
    2-3 garlic cloves, minced
    1 heaping tsp. grated ginger root
    1 tsp. Thai curry paste (available
        at Asian stores or grocery
        stores)
    1 Tbsp. vegetable oil

Sauté the above if desired, then add:
1 cup chickpeas, soaked overnight in water
1 piece of lemon grass or lemon peel
2-3 lime leaves
1 can coconut milk

Fill crockpot almost full with water. Turn crockpot on low and cook for 3-8 hours. Taste and adjust seasoning.

Serve topped with chopped coriander and rice noodles.

VIETNAMESE RICE PAPER ROLLS

These are quick, easy, and tasty for a light summer lunch or beginning course for dinner.

>   12 round (8-9") or 24 square (6") rice paper wrappers
>   (from Chinese or Thai store)
>   6-8 leaves romaine, Chinese cabbage, or spinach, cut into
>   very thin strips
>   1 cup mung bean sprouts
>   1 large carrot, julienned or grated
>   1/2 cup cilantro leaves
>   1/2 cup mint leaves
>   1 cup firm or smoked tofu, cut into thin strips
>   1/4 cup minced peanuts
>   Spicy peanut sauce or sweet and sour dipping sauce

Fill a pie plate with lukewarm water. Have a roll of paper towels handy. Dip a rice paper wrapper in water for 2-5 seconds, then place on dinner plate and cover with damp paper towel. Repeat with rest of wrappers, finishing with a paper towel. In a bowl, combine greens, bean sprouts, carrot, herbs, tofu, and peanuts. Add about 1/2 cup spicy peanut sauce and toss gently. Remove rice paper wrappers one at a time and place on flat surface. Place filling (3 Tbsp. for small wrappers, 1/3 cup for large) on half wrapper closest to you. Roll up tightly, folding sides in, and put on plate. When all rolls are made, serve immediately with dipping sauce or cover tightly with plastic wrap and store in refrigerator until serving time. They will keep up to one day. To serve, cut rolls in half, garnish with cilantro, and pass extra sauces.

SWEET AND SOUR DIPPING SAUCE
1/2 cup rice vinegar
1/2 cup honey
1/2 tsp. salt
2 Tbsp. chopped cilantro
3 Tbsp. chopped roasted peanuts
1 tsp. chopped red onion
1 tsp. (or to taste) minced chili

Heat vinegar until warm. Add honey to dissolve. Cool and add cilantro, chili, and onion. Add peanuts just before serving. (Makes about 1 1/3 cups.)

C.J.'S SPICY PEANUT SAUCE
1 onion, minced
1 clove garlic, minced
1" piece ginger, minced
1 Tbsp. roasted sesame oil
Sauté above together until soft.

Add:
2 Tbsp. peanut butter
1 Tbsp. soy sauce
1 Tbsp. brown sugar or dried cane juice
1 Tbsp. chutney
1 tsp. curry powder
1 cup of water or coconut milk
Simmer for 20-30 minutes, then add:
Juice of 1/2 lemon

Taste and adjust seasonings.
Serve as a dipping sauce for rice paper or egg rolls, on steamed or sautéed vegetables, rice, or cooked rice noodles.

DR. FRY'S SUPER SOY SHAKE
1/2 cup soy milk
1/3 cup tofu, soft
3 Tbsp. soy powder
1 Tbsp. flaxseeds, ground in coffee grinder
1/2 cup to 1 cup juice (e.g., apple, orange, grapefruit)
Fresh fruit, such as bananas, strawberries, and peaches.
Calcium powder (1,000-1,500mg) may be added for
    additional nutrition.

Mix all ingredients in blender and enjoy!
Most of the ingredients for this recipe may
be purchased at local health food stores.

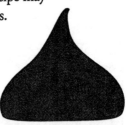

BITTERSWEET CHOCOLATE/BANANA MOUSSE
1 cup semisweet chocolate chips
1 10-oz. box of soft silken tofu
2 large ripe bananas
1 tsp. vanilla extract
2 to 3 Tbsp. brown sugar

Melt chocolate chips in a double boiler. In the meantime, puree
one banana and the tofu in a blender. Add remaining banana in
chunks along with the vanilla, sugar, and a pinch of salt. Pour in
melted chocolate and puree until completely smooth. Transfer to
large serving dish or individual dishes and chill for at least two hours.

Lifestyle tips that won't fail you

Some of your everyday habits could be harming your health and making your menopausal symptoms worse. What you are doing—or *not* doing—could also be putting you at risk for serious illness.

Here is our eight-point lifestyle modification plan:

1. **If you smoke, quit.** This recommendation is worth repeating. In the United States, more than 140,000 women die each year from smoking-related diseases. In addition to cancer and heart disease, smoking worsens menopausal symptoms and contributes to osteoporosis. Women who smoke typically experience menopause at an earlier age than women who don't.

2. **Control stress.** We recognize that it is not always possible to control stress entirely in today's fast-paced society. However, you must make an effort to reduce the stress in your life. Utilize calming herbal teas (e.g., chamomile, valerian), breathing techniques, regular massage, and yoga to get the stress in your life under control. Stress can weaken the immune system, increase your risk of heart disease, trigger mental/emotional problems, and exacerbate menopausal symptoms in most women. Stress is hard on the adrenal glands, which are the main source of hormone production after menopause.

3. **Meditation.** Hundreds of scientific studies have documented the beneficial effects of meditation on physical, emotional, and spiritual health. Meditation reduces the production of cortisol, the "fight-or-flight" hormone associated with chronic stress. Meditation lowers blood pressure, and cholesterol levels, and may help reverse heart disease. In his book, *Reversing Heart Disease*, Dr. Dean Ornish writes that just 20 minutes each day in silent prayer and meditation provides a wealth of benefits for the body, mind, and spirit.

4. Be positive. Surround yourself with optimistic, supportive people. Focus on the positive things happening in your life and search for ways to find joy, peace, and happiness. Science has confirmed a direct link between our thoughts and our health. An upbeat attitude will help you control irritating symptoms and prevent illness.

5. Laugh often. We are not encouraging you to giggle uncontrollably during your next meeting at work. However, we urge you to get your fair share of hearty "belly laughs" each day. Laughter is good for the mind, the soul, and the menopausal woman.

6. Nurture your spirit. Be kind to yourself and pay attention to your needs. As women, we often spend most of our lives caring for others, while we neglect our own needs. Pay attention to your spirit. Menopause is a great time to identify what you need and want out of life. Be sure not only to give, but also remain open to receiving love—you deserve it and your well-being depends on it.

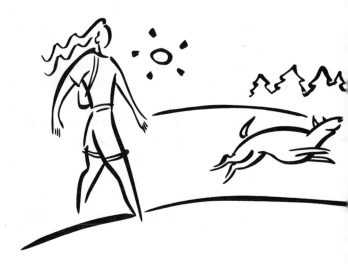

7. **Continue to grow.** Work at stimulating the student within you. Studies have shown that the "use-it-or-lose-it" maxim applies to the mind as well as the body. Find ways to make your life journey one of constant learning and discovery.

8. **Be physical.** Here's another recommendation worth repeating. Physical activity is your key to lifelong optimal health and vitality. Consistent exercise appears to be the real "fountain of youth."

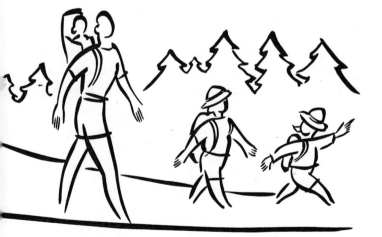

The healing powers of physical activity

The scientific community has demonstrated that physical activity is the closest thing we've got to a cure-all. No pill can come close to matching the power of this panacea.

The benefits of exercise include:
- reduced menopausal symptoms;
- reduced depression, stress, and anxiety;
- weight maintenance or weight loss;
- decreased risk of heart disease;
- enhanced immunity and reduced risk of some cancers;
- reduced risk of osteoporosis;
- reduced risk of diabetes;
- improved sleep;
- enhanced self-image and elevated mood; and
- increased strength and mobility.

Aside from all the clinical data, we have found in our practice that patients who exercise tend to have far fewer problems getting through menopause. Unfortunately, too many women are not exercising. The National Institutes of Health recommends light to moderate exercise for at least 30 minutes a day six days a week. Consistency, rather than intensity, is the important factor here. Every woman needs to make exercise a regular part of her weekly routine.

Note: If you have been inactive for a long period of time, are extremely overweight, or have specific health problems that may worsen with physical activity, consult your doctor before beginning an exercise program.

Chapter Four

Using herbs that heal

Since the dawn of time, plants have been used to heal and rejuvenate both body and soul. For as long as there have been herbs, there have been herbal medicines. Many researchers believe that these powerful, traditional medicines will become invaluable health tools in the near future. In our clinical practices, the future is already here.

As healthcare practitioners, we are not alone in our enthusiasm for herbal medicines. The sales of herbal supplements in the United States exceeded $4 billion in 1999. While the herbal market has grown rapidly in recent years, the public is closely scrutinizing the quality of available products. They are seeking an assurance of consistent high quality, efficacy, and safety.

After the Dietary Supplement Health and Education Act (DSHEA) passed in 1994, manufacturers, experts in nutrition and botanicals, and legislators started working in a conscientious alliance with consumers at the grassroots level. DSHEA defines dietary supplements, places the responsibility for their safety on manufacturers, and identifies how literature may be used in connection with sales. Furthermore, DSHEA created an Office of Dietary Supplements (ODS) in the National Institutes of Health (NIH). This came with a mandate to coordinate scientific research relating to dietary supplements within NIH, and to advise federal agencies on issues concerning dietary supplements and herbs.

There is a great deal of motivation to continue these lines of research. James A. Duke, Ph.D., herbalist, author, and retired researcher with the USDA, states: "As study results become publicized, these botanical alternatives will become more attractive to the intelligent American consumer. I predict that Americans will finally have had enough of the side effects of synthetic drugs…they will return to the ancestral medicines that their genes have known for more than two million years."

The vast amount of research available on herbs has stimulated a groundswell of support and a resurgence of interest in this form of treatment. Consumers are encouraged to choose a high-quality product, which was produced using good manufacturing practices (GMPs) and is appropriately standardized for its key compound(s).

Herbs have been shown to ease a wide variety of conditions and can be used as both preventive medicine and effective treatment. Menopause is one of the conditions that normally responds well to herbal medicines.

Herbal supplements are different than synthesized pharmaceuticals. Various constituents in herbs work synergistically to address several disease factors. To ensure the quality of products, industries are using GMPs, which ensure strict quality control.

Herbs for menopause

Why do menopausal women respond so successfully to herbal medicine? We feel it is because an herbal approach is more natural—the various constituents in herbs gently and synergistically work with a woman's body to promote balance and harmony. In fact, we do not believe that menopause is a "condition" at all. It is a natural life process.

There was a time, not too long ago, when menopause was considered an "estrogen deficiency." Women were told this was a time of irreversible and inevitable physical and mental decline. Today, we know this is not true. Menopause is really a new beginning on a different path.

As with all new directions in life, some transitions are smoother than others. For example, if you've had a child, you may recall a difficult or an easy pregnancy. If you've changed careers, you may have felt invigorated or petrified. During those times, you found ways to support yourself (body and soul) during the change.

Herbs can provide powerful support during your menopausal transition. What we have found most appealing about this approach is the synergistic effect that results from combining various herbs. In other words, the combined impact is greater than the sum of their individual effects.

We found a specific combination of herbs to be very beneficial. We have chosen these herbs because they contain important components that provide a balancing effect. These herbs have also been shown to be effective *and* safe.

The reason these herbs are so useful for menopause is that many of them contain phytoestrogens. Phytoestrogens have a normalizing effect. They work in cases of estrogen dominance, characterized by fibroids, fibrocystic breast disease, and PMS. They also work when the body is not producing enough estrogen, as in the

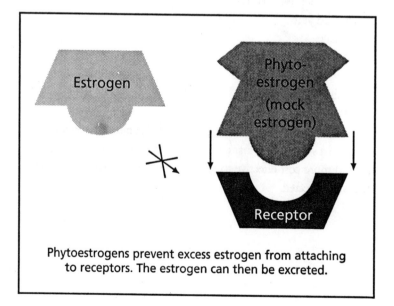

Phytoestrogens prevent excess estrogen from attaching to receptors. The estrogen can then be excreted.

case of menopause. While phytoestrogens mimic estrogens, they are 1/400th as potent as synthetic estrogens.

For menopausal symptoms, we have found that phytoestrogen-containing herbs offer significant advantages over conventionally prescribed estrogen. Although estrogens may pose significant health risks, including an increased risk of cancer, gallbladder disease, and stroke, phytoestrogens are not associated with these side effects.

Foreign estrogens, known as xenoestrogens, come from hormones in chickens, herbicides, pesticides, and other environmental or food sources. They may mimic estrogens in the human body. However, because they are foreign substances, these estrogens do not fit perfectly into the body's estrogen receptor sites. They can actually make menopausal symptoms worse, or may contribute to cancer and other illnesses.

Natural phytoestrogens are a better fit. They also help block foreign estrogens from attaching to the receptor sites, so the body can easily get rid of them.

The following herbs are profiled in this section:
- black cohosh
- soybean isoflavones
- wild yam
- sage
- chastetree berry
- vervain
- astragalus
- motherwort

While these herbs can be purchased separately, we recommend you find a supplement that contains all of them. This will make it easier and more cost-effective to take the herbs every day. Use it consistently, as directed.

Phytoestrogens and cancer

The relationship between phytoestrogens and cancer has generated some heated controversy. Many experts claim that phytoestrogens protect against cancer. Others caution that phytoestrogens can contribute to cancer; specifically, estrogen-dependent cancers such as breast cancer. Maureen Miller Pelletier, M.D., an expert in women's health issues, states that, "Epidemiological studies show that soy consumption is associated with a lowered risk of breast cancer, lung cancer, leukemia, and prostate cancer." Soy foods, such as tofu, contain phytoestrogens.

Jesse Lynn Hanley, M.D., a clinician who specializes in women's health, urges women with a family history of breast cancer to seek relief from menopausal symptoms, but to be cautious. She advises patients to first make dietary and lifestyle changes, including incorporating soy foods into their diet. If patients do not respond to these changes, she says, "I introduce weaker estrogens and avoid the highly standardized forms of black cohosh and red clover presently on the market."

Mark Messina, Ph.D., an expert in nutrition, states, "The issue of whether women who've had estrogen-dependent breast cancers should take soy is certainly controversial. Experts disagree on what advice to give. Some data suggest that soy may exert estrogenic effects on breast tissue, whereas other data suggest soy may benefit women with and without breast cancer. The epidemiologic data suggest that soy consumption is protective. Personally, I think caution is appropriate."

Clearly, more research is needed on the impact of phytoestrogens on women at high risk of breast cancer. Soy foods and phytoestrogens, taken at the recommended dosages, seem to be safe for this patient population. Certainly, herbs are safer than conventionally prescribed estrogen for women who have had breast cancer, or have a strong family history of breast cancer. Women in Asian countries traditionally eat soy-based foods every day, and their breast cancer risk is very low.

If you are concerned about taking prescription estrogen, discuss your options with your physician.

A word about standardization

Some herbal extracts provide the most benefit when they are standardized. These products are made by extracting beneficial constituents to create a solid extract that can be put into a capsule or tablet. Advanced scientific techniques make it possible to identify an isolated compound or compounds that have the most therapeutic impact within many plants.

"Standardization ensures that each capsule has the same amount of therapeutic activity," according to *Buyer Be Wise: The Consumer's Guide to Buying Quality Nutritional Supplements,* by Karolyn A. Gazella.

Since herbs contain many compounds and vary by nature, standardization with markers is important. Through standardization, consumers can be assured they are receiving a high-quality product that will produce consistent results.

Herbalist Dr. James Duke makes another good point about standardization in *Buyer Be Wise*: "Accurate measurement of active constituents allows the herbal extract to be duplicated again and again, assuring consistent potency in every batch..."

Standardization provides the most potent, consistent health benefits with herbs that have identifiable active compounds. Of the herbs featured in this book, we feel the following should be standardized:

- black cohosh
- soybean isoflavones
- wild yam

Black cohosh

Black cohosh (*Cimicifuga racemosa*) is native to the United States and Canada. This perennial plant grows up to five feet tall and prefers shady woods with rich, deep soil. The root of the black cohosh plant is used for its medicinal qualities and is, not surprisingly, black.

Native Americans, and then eclectic physicians of the late 1800s and early 1900s, traditionally used black cohosh for its anti-inflammatory and sedative qualities. It was primarily used to treat female complaints, including painful menstrual cramping, delayed periods, mastitis (i.e., inflammation of the breast, usually due to infection), ovarian pain, menopausal symptoms (e.g., hot flashes, night sweats, vaginal dryness, and depression), and false or true labor pains. In addition to high blood pressure and tinnitus (i.e., ringing in the ears), black cohosh was also used for nerve and muscle pain in conditions such as neuralgia, rheumatism, arthritis, and headaches.

Effects of black cohosh

Symptom	% no longer present	% improved	Total % improved
Hot flashes	43.3	43.3	86.6
Profuse perspiration	49.9	38.6	88.5
Headache	45.7	36.2	81.9
Vertigo	51.6	35.2	86.8
Heart palpitation	54.6	35.2	89.8
Ringing in ears	54.8	38.1	92.9
Nervousness/irritability	42.4	43.2	85.6
Sleep disturbances	46.1	30.7	76.8
Depressive moods	46.0	36.5	82.5
(Stolze, 1982)			

Within the last 40 years, scientific research has confirmed these benefits. In 1960, Dr. Brucker, a German physician, published a four-year study involving 517 women who used black cohosh extract to relieve menopausal symptoms. Dr. Brucker recorded a number of benefits and no side effects. Since that time, several solid clinical studies have confirmed that black cohosh can effectively alleviate menopausal mood swings, depression, anxiety, fatigue, hot flashes, and vaginal dryness.

The prestigious German Commission E (the medical council that analyzes herbal medicines in Germany) has documented the clinical value of black cohosh. This is considered the most extensively studied herb for menopause available today.

One large study of black cohosh featured 629 menopausal women. Most of the participants noticed improvements in their symptoms within four weeks. Within eight weeks, a large percentage of the study participants reported complete relief of their menopausal symptoms.

According to Mark Stengler, N.D., author and naturopathic physician, "Clinical studies involving more than 1,700 patients, over a three- to six-month period, showed excellent tolerance of black cohosh."

When taken at the recommended dosage, black cohosh is a very safe herb. A small number of women have reported occasional stomach upset or digestive disturbances. Taking the herb with food, or combining it with the herb vervain, helps alleviate this potential side effect. Vervain is very soothing to the stomach. The herb astragalus also complements black cohosh.

Historically, black cohosh has been used at the end of pregnancy to induce stronger, more efficient uterine contractions. However, we do not recommend this or most other herbs for women who are pregnant or lactating.

Soybean isoflavones

Soybeans are the richest food source of a type of phytoestrogen called isoflavones. These isoflavones have been studied extensively and have demonstrated a number of health benefits, including relief of menopausal symptoms.

After being introduced to soybeans in England, Ben Franklin was so impressed that he brought them back to the United States. Until fairly recently, soybeans were primarily used as livestock feed. Today, media attention on the many health benefits of soy has made this unassuming little bean quite popular.

Asians typically consume plenty of soy-based foods such as tofu, edamame, soy milk, tempeh, miso, and soy sauce. Studies have shown that they have a much lower rate of heart disease and cancers of the breast, colon, and prostate. Asian women also have far fewer menopausal complaints than North American women.

Some epidemiological studies (i.e., population studies) have shown that when Asian women adopt the typical North American diet, their risk of breast cancer increases to the level of other North American women.

Soy isoflavones not only help ease menopausal symptoms, they also help prevent the three conditions menopausal women are most concerned about: cancer, heart disease, and osteoporosis.

Unfortunately, many women tend to shy away from soy foods because they are unaccustomed to the taste and texture. Although soy foods are the best source of isoflavones, this is a legitimate concern. Nutritional supplements that contain soy isoflavones provide an option for women who do not eat soy foods. Another option is to "bury" soy protein powder or tofu into convenient shakes and other recipes. Even if you do decide to use a nutritional supplement with soy isoflavones, adding soy to the diet will provide further health benefits. Try out the tasty recipes we've included on pages 20 through 24.

Soy isoflavones have been shown to be very safe. According to registered dietician and nutritional counselor Patti Tveit Milligan, M.S., R.D. "In Japan, the average person consumes 20 to 100mg of isoflavones per day from soy foods. It has been suggested that 50mg daily or more of isoflavones would be prudent to consume through soy foods and/or a concentrated soy supplement."

The only reason you may not want to incorporate more soy into your diet is the possibility of a soy allergy. Keep in mind, however, that if you have this allergy, you can work with a food allergy specialist to overcome it.

Wild yam

The wild yam (*Dioscorea villosa*) plant is native to North and Central America. This perennial climbing vine can grow up to 20 feet. The root of the plant is the part used for medicinal purposes.

Historically, wild yam was used to treat menstrual disorders, miscarriage, infertility, endometriosis, and symptoms of menopause. More recently, wild yam became popular when it was believed that one of its active components, diosgenin, could be converted into progesterone in the body. Some manufacturers still claim that wild yam creams are the same as progesterone creams, but we now know that the body cannot change diosgenin into progesterone. Although wild yam is not a replacement for progesterone, it does provide a wide variety of significant therapeutic benefits.

The significant antioxidant activity of wild yam makes it beneficial for the heart. Research indicates that wild yam can reduce "bad" (LDL) cholesterol while increasing "good" (HDL) cholesterol. In addition, wild yam has been used to reduce inflammation and relieve spasmodic pain in the digestive tract, female reproductive tract, and muscles. It is also considered a natural treatment for gallbladder inflammation, which often plagues older women.

Chinese herbal medicine considers wild yam to be a "yin tonic" that supports the body's energy production, as well as adrenal and thyroid function. It is often recommended for symptoms of fatigue, hypothyroidism, excessive sweating, frequent urination, and weak digestion.

Supporting the adrenal glands is extremely important during the early stages of menopause. The adrenal glands take over for the ovaries in producing androstenedione, which is converted to estrone in the fat, liver, and kidneys. Estrone is the dominant estrogen in postmenopausal women. Estrone is about 12 times weaker than estradiol, the most potent of estrogens, but it can still help alleviate menopausal symptoms. That's why optimal adrenal function is important during perimenopause/menopause. In addition to supporting adrenal function with herbs, reducing stress will help.

No side effects or adverse reactions have been reported when wild yam extract is used as directed. Very large amounts of wild yam may cause nausea.

Sage

The Latin name for sage is *Salvia officinalis.* Salvia is taken from the Latin word, *salvare,* which means "to cure." This aromatic cooking spice has a long history of varied uses, including anti-aging and memory enhancement.

The sage plant grows as a bush up to two feet high. It has an erect woody stem and oblong greenish-gray or purple leaves that are one to three inches long. These leaves are the parts of the plant most often used; however, all of the parts above ground have demonstrated both medical and aromatic qualities.

Sage is a powerful antioxidant, which could explain its many health-promoting benefits. It also relieves menopausal symptoms. For example, sage has anti-hidrotic properties, which means it can stop sweating. The estrogen-like effects of sage make it ideal for alleviating hot flashes and night sweats. In addition, it is considered a tonic medicine that enhances digestion and calms the nerves.

Recent research with sage has focused on its antioxidant properties. Sage is believed to be an anti-aging medicine because it helps reduce the effects of free-radical damage associated with aging. Perhaps that explains the proverb from medieval times: "Why should a man die while sage grows in his garden?"

Sage is a perfect herb to add to your menopause herbal supplement program. Sage is also safe, although it is not recommended for pregnant or lactating women. According to the German Commission E, sage is not known to negatively interact with other herbs or drugs.

Chastetree berry

Also known as *Vitex agnus-castus*, the chastetree is actually a small shrub with violet flowers shaped like fingers. It is native to the Mediterranean and western Asia. The small black dried berries are the part of the plant used medicinally.

In addition to a long history of use, clinical studies over the past 40 years have shown that chastetree berries help balance estrogen and progesterone levels. They do this by influencing the hypothalamus and the pituitary gland, which in turn helps normalize FSH and LH production. Chastetree berries specifically work to increase LH. For this reason, it is one of the most commonly prescribed herbs in Europe for the treatment of perimenopausal symptoms.

Because chastetree berries help stabilize fluctuating female hormone levels, chastetree berry extract can help a variety of conditions, including:

- premenstrual syndrome (PMS);
- cyclical breast swelling;
- amenorrhea (i.e., absence of menstruation);
- hormonal acne;
- fibrocystic breasts; and
- irregular or heavy menstrual bleeding.

In addition, chastetree berry extract helps control symptoms associated with menopause, including hot flashes, dizziness, loss of libido, vaginal dryness, and depression.

Side effects associated with chastetree berry extract are rare. It is safe and non-toxic when taken at recommended dosages. In clinical studies, only one percent of participants reported side effects. These included slight headaches and occasional skin rashes. Although *The PDR for Herbal Medicine* cautions against its use for women who are

lactating, chastetree berries have been used in Europe to increase lac-
tation for women who cannot generate sufficient breast milk.

This herb is not recommended for children or pregnant women.
There are no known interactions with drugs or other herbs.

Chastetree berry extract does not work quickly. It must be
taken for several cycles to achieve optimum benefit. If taken over a
period of six to nine months, the results will be long-lasting and are
worth the wait.

Vervain

While we haven't heard much about vervain (*Verbena officinalis*)
in the mainstream media, it is another herb that has been used
throughout history. In Egypt, vervain was included in love potions
and dedicated to Isis, the goddess of fertility.

Although vervain was primarily native to the Mediterranean
areas, it now grows wild throughout much of the world, including
the United States. It is a perennial plant that stands about 30 to 60
centimeters high, with erect wiry stems and oblong, deeply toothed
leaves. All of the parts of the plant above ground are considered
medicinal.

Traditionally, herbalists have used vervain as a nervous system
tonic to calm frayed nerves and to ease tension, headaches, insomnia,
and depression. Homeopathic medicine recommends vervain for
mental stress and the inability to relax. Its bitter principles have
been shown to enhance digestion and stimulate the liver, thereby
promoting the elimination of excess hormones. Both the *PDR for
Herbal Medicine* and the *German Commission E* cite its benefits for
menopausal symptoms, as well as nervous disorders, fatigue, and
digestive and gallbladder complaints. It can also be used as a gargle
for sore throats.

No precautions or adverse effects are indicated for vervain
when taken at the recommended dosages. Pregnant women should
avoid taking vervain. In large dosages, vervain can induce vomiting.

Astragalus

While you may not have heard of this important herb, astragalus (*Astragalus membranaceus*) has been used in China as a tonic for thousands of years. It is finally gaining popularity in North America. This perennial plant is native to eastern China and Mongolia. It grows up to two feet, and its leaves are divided into 12 to 18 leaflets in a feather-like arrangement.

As an overall body tonic, astragalus plays many important roles. It promotes adrenal function, helps the body cope with stress, and supports the immune system. In addition, recent studies have shown that it benefits the heart. All these functions, of course, are important to the menopausal woman.

According to California herbalist and author Kathi Keville, astragalus is not only an immune-system stimulator, but also a heart tonic that helps prevent and treat arrhythmia (i.e., irregular heartbeat). Many studies have shown that it stabilizes blood pressure and protects against lipid peroxidation, a process that can damage the heart. In addition, astragalus has been shown to improve memory.

Many other studies have focused primarily on astragalus's ability to stimulate the immune system, warding off the common cold and other viruses. Animal studies have demonstrated specific immune-enhancing capabilities: Astragalus triggers T-cell activity and stimulates macrophages, immune cells that consume foreign material. In studies at the National Cancer Institute, along with five other cancer research institutes, astragalus has been shown to boost a depressed immune system in both cancer patients and healthy study participants.

Astragalus is an extremely mild but deep-acting herbal medicine. There are no known side effects or contraindications. Some herbalists do not recommend astragalus during an acute fever because of its inherent "warming nature."

Motherwort

The last in our series of herbs for menopause is motherwort. This perennial plant is native to central Asia. However, it has now been naturalized in most of Europe and North America. You will often see it growing wild along the roadside and in forest areas. The herb's Latin name is *Leonurus cardiaca*. In Greek this means "lion's tail," and appropriately describes the shaggy, deeply toothed leaves that hang from the plant.

Motherwort has been used historically for female reproductive conditions, the last stages of pregnancy/labor, and as a heart tonic. In 1652, herbalist Nicholas Culpepper wrote about motherwort, "there is no better herb to drive away melancholy vapors from the heart, to strengthen it, and make the mind cheerful."

Herbalists have traditionally used motherwort as a tonic for the heart, specifically in cases of anxiety or nervous tension that result in palpitations and arrhythmias. It has been shown to actually promote relaxation without causing drowsiness.

Because many women notice increased heart palpitations during menopause, motherwort is an ideal herb. In addition, motherwort helps stabilize blood-vessel sensitivity to fluctuating estrogen levels and protects against heart disease. Animal studies have also shown that it can lower blood pressure.

Furthermore, this soothing herb can help ease anxiety and insomnia, two key menopausal complaints. Motherwort has also been used to help alleviate painful, spasmodic, or delayed menstrual periods. Some herbalists use it during the last week of pregnancy or during labor to help facilitate proper contractions.

Motherwort has no known side effects, contraindications, or interactions with other drugs or herbs when used at the proper dosage. Because it can stimulate the uterine lining, it should not be used during heavy menstrual bleeding. It should only be used during the last week of pregnancy or during labor under the direct supervision of a qualified healthcare professional. Women who are lactating should not use motherwort.

Chapter Five

Frequently asked questions

Following are questions that women frequently ask about menopause:

Q: **My doctor prescribed low-dose birth control pills for my perimenopausal symptoms, which include night sweats and mood swings. I have a history of breast tenderness and the birth control pills make the pain even worse. Is there a more natural alternative that can relieve my symptoms without the side effects of birth control pills?**

A: Absolutely. The smooth transition program outlined in this book can help alleviate night sweats and mood swings. Because this program uses natural substances, it is much gentler and free of the side effects of birth control pills.

For best results, wean yourself off the birth control pills as you begin the program. Many women can stop taking birth control pills "cold turkey," without any problem. Some women are more comfortable doing it gradually; i.e., taking a birth control pill every other day for one month, then every three days the next month.

If you're taking birth control pills to prevent pregnancy, you can continue to take them along with a menopause herbal formula. Many of our patients take both, and we have never seen any contraindications. However, if you're taking birth control pills for endometriosis, fibroids, or breast tenderness, you may be able to discontinue them two or three months after you start taking the herbal formula. Because herbs work more gradually, it may take two or three months before the natural menopause formula successfully relieves your symptoms.

Note: If you discontinue birth control pills, and you wish to avoid pregnancy, make sure you are using another effective birth control method.

If you've taken the menopause herbal formula for a month or two, and still experience breast tenderness, we recommend chastetree berry (*Vitex agnus-castus*) extract. Take two capsules twice a day for a month, and cut down to one capsule twice a day after that. Within two to three months, you probably won't need it anymore. Another option is to rub in 1/4 teaspoon of progesterone cream for 25 days a month, then stop for five days. It may take two or three months for the progesterone to help your system adjust.

Finally, eliminating caffeine from your diet may help relieve lumpy, sore breasts.

Q: What exactly is progesterone cream? Can it relieve symptoms of perimenopause?

A: Progesterone is a hormone that stimulates changes in the lining of the uterus to nourish a developing embryo. When progesterone is produced, estrogen levels drop. Shifts in hormonal balance can often affect mood. A progesterone cream can help restore hormonal balance and improve symptoms related to hormonal imbalance, such as premenstrual syndrome (PMS), perimenopause, and menopause. In addition, scientific studies demonstrate that progesterone promotes bone strength.

Progesterone is more quickly and easily absorbed in the cream form. This form also allows you to control your dosages according to your needs. Often, a 10 to 30mg daily dose is enough to relieve PMS-related irritability or anxiety.

Q: **I'm confused about vitamins. I am experiencing many symptoms associated with menopause, including hot flashes and mood swings. Which vitamins should I take?**

A: In addition to a complete daily multivitamin/mineral product, you should consider taking 400 IU of vitamin E. A complete bone formula, containing calcium, magnesium, boron, vitamin D, and vitamin K, will help prevent osteoporosis. Also, if you are feeling stressed, a vitamin B complex may help.

Q: **I am still menstruating, but my periods are irregular and I am experiencing hot flashes and mood swings. I didn't think this would begin until after my periods stopped. What can I do to relieve these symptoms?**

A: You are probably experiencing perimenopause. Although you are still menstruating, your levels of estrogen and progesterone are declining, creating an imbalance and resulting in menopausal symptoms. The smooth transition program is not only useful for menopause; it can also help women who are experiencing perimenopause.

Q: My doctor put me on conventional hormone therapy, but I'd like to switch to a more natural program. Do you have any recommendations on how to go about this?

A: First, we encourage you to consult a knowledgeable herbalist or naturopath. To find a qualified practitioner in your area, call the American Holistic Medical Association at (703) 556-9728.

When we have patients who want to switch, we slowly wean them off conventional hormones. Every three weeks, they decrease their pills by one a week. It takes three or four months to stop completely.

In the meantime, these women start taking a menopausal herbal formula. They also begin to apply 1/2 teaspoon of progesterone cream twice a day for 25 days, then off for five days. In addition, we also recommend that they add more soy to their diet. Drinking sage tea before bedtime can help alleviate night sweats.

Keep in mind that a menopausal herbal formula is not as strong as conventional hormone replacement therapy (HRT). It doesn't work as quickly. In addition, it often takes more effort to follow a natural program than to pop a pill and forget about it. However, a natural program doesn't have the side effects associated with HRT. It is better for your health, and better for your peace of mind.

Chapter Six

The smooth transition plan

While it may be difficult to believe at times, menopause is a perfect opportunity for a new beginning, filled with hope, contentment, and fulfillment. This can become your time to tap into a new form of creative energy. It can be a time to focus on the big picture while learning to enjoy life's little pleasures. Patients often tell us that once they get their menopausal symptoms under control, they experience a sense of renewal. Our smooth transition plan helps relieve the discomforts of menopause, so you can experience the positive aspects of this change.

Before beginning any new health program, we recommend that our patients learn as much as they can about their options. The information you gather will help you develop an individualized plan. This information will allow you to work with your healthcare practitioner to obtain optimal health and well being.

Keep in mind that this is a process. Chances are, it won't happen overnight. Be patient with yourself and others. Be especially attuned to the messages your body is sending you. Get to know your body and learn how to read your individual road signs. Utilize the same powerful intuition that has helped you be a good mother, partner, friend, or manager, to help you achieve balance and harmony in your life.

The 90/10 rule

Your diet and lifestyle will determine the success of your smooth transition into menopause. Making healthful diet and lifestyle choices are the most critical factors in our smooth transition strategy.

Consider the components of your diet as tools you can use to achieve your health goals. Avoid choices that lead you away from your health goals. The same is true for lifestyle factors. Smoking, drinking too much alcohol, or being negative are all choices. Steer clear of choices that disrupt your health. Instead, focus on activities that enhance your health.

Naturally, this is easier said than done. That's why we recommend the 90/10 rule. Simply put, the 90/10 rule suggests that you choose the healthy path 90 percent of the time. That way, if you fall off the "health wagon" 10 percent of the time, the consequences are negligible.

Most of us are still working toward that 90 percent. Don't be too hard on yourself if you cannot reach that percentage right away. Give yourself time. Many of the diet and lifestyle recommendations in this book may be dramatic for some people. Take small steps toward your ultimate goal. You'll be surprised how quickly you are able to make the healthy choice 90 percent of the time.

Journaling can help

Putting your feelings down on paper is a great way to vent frustrations and let yourself dream. Keeping a journal is something you can do just for you. The words you write and the thoughts you convey are for your eyes only. Nobody will criticize or judge you.

Journaling is a great way to get to know yourself. It allows you to take an inner journey and let all your feelings come out on paper. And best of all, it's easy. All you need to get started is a notebook, pen, and some time each week (or day, if you can). Some journaling experts even recommend having colored pens and crayons handy in case you get the urge to draw how you are feeling.

Here are some general guidelines for keeping a journal:

- **Be consistent.** Writing in a journal several times a week will help make this activity a part of your routine.
- **Stay in order.** Date the first page of each journal entry so you can keep a chronological order of your thoughts and feelings.
- **Choose an appropriate place.** Journaling requires some quiet time in a relaxing, comfortable place with no interruptions or distractions. Soft music that gives you a feeling of peace and serenity may enhance your journal experience.
- **Just keep writing.** Remember, this journal is for your eyes only. Do not edit or think too much prior to writing. Just let the thoughts flow. This is not homework. Make this a pleasurable, creative experience.

Sometimes making lists can help capture thoughts or get the process going. Here are some lists that we suggest you start with:

- **List all the things for which you are grateful.** This is known as a gratitude journal and women have reported that such a journal has virtually changed their attitude and life perspective.
- **List all the positive qualities you possess.** This is ideal for women who suffer from a low self-image.
- **List all your life's accomplishments.** You will be surprised at how full your life has been.
- **List all your goals.** This is a time to really let yourself go. We prefer to think of this as a dream list; however, you must believe that these dreams can come true.

You will be amazed at how much these lists reveal. Journaling is another way to nurture yourself during menopause. It is also an excellent tool for recording your symptoms and your responses to the changes you make as part of your smooth transition program.

Herbal review

Herbal remedies can provide powerful relief and support during the menopausal transition. For this reason, herbal extracts are considered an important part of our smooth transition program. Let's summarize the herbs we've featured in this book.

Black cohosh:

- Relieves menopause-related hot flashes, depression, and vaginal dryness.
- Beneficial for painful menstruation and delayed periods.
- Studied extensively in Europe.
- No known contraindications or negative interactions with drugs or other herbs.
- Side effects include occasional stomach upset.

Soybean isoflavones:

- Relieves menopausal symptoms.
- Studies suggest that isoflavones protect against some cancers and strengthen bones.
- No known contraindications or negative interactions with drugs or other herbs.
- No known side effects.

Wild yam:

- Antispasmodic, relieves spasms in the female reproductive tract and gallbladder.
- Antioxidant activity protects the heart and lowers cholesterol.
- Supports adrenal and thyroid function and is recommended for tiredness, excessive sweating, and frequent urination.
- No known side effects or adverse reactions when used at the recommended dosage.

Sage:
- Alleviates sweating and hot flashes.
- Has calming properties.
- Powerful antioxidant believed to promote longevity and improve memory.
- Not known to interact negatively with other herbs or drugs.

Chastetree berry:
- Among the most commonly prescribed herbs in Europe for the treatment of perimenopausal symptoms.
- The hormonal action stimulates follicle-stimulating hormones (FSH), increases luteinizing hormones (LH), and balances estrogen to alleviate symptoms of menopause.
- Not known to work quickly; usually takes as long as six to nine months.
- Extremely safe and nontoxic.

Vervain:
- Nervous system tonic that calms the nerves, eases tension, and relieves headaches and insomnia.
- Treats fatigue and digestive and gallbladder complaints.
- Safe at recommended dosages.
- In large dosages, it can cause vomiting.

Astragalus:
- Stimulates the immune system.
- Promotes heart health.
- Supports the adrenal glands and relieves stress.
- Extremely mild, yet deep-acting herb.
- No known side effects or contraindications.

Motherwort:
- Primarily used for heart complaints associated with anxiety or nervous tension, such as palpitations and arrhythmias.
- Promotes relaxation without causing drowsiness.
- Helps relieve anxiety-induced insomnia.
- Eases painful, spasmodic, or delayed menstruation.
- No known side effects or contraindications.
- Should not be used during heavy menstrual bleeding.

General warning:
- Do not take if pregnant or breastfeeding, or if contemplating a pregnancy in the near future. Consult with a health professional if you are taking birth control pills or other prescription medications.

Final thoughts

We hope you find this book helpful. Please share it with a friend who may also be suffering needlessly with menopausal symptoms. Our goal is to touch the lives of as many women as possible. There is no need to suffer when you go through menopause naturally. We wish you a smooth transition.

Resources

<u>INTERNET</u>

- healthy.com = the most comprehensive source of independent natural health information.

- holisticmedicine.com = the web site of the American Holistic Medical Association, with information on where to find a holistic physician.

- impakt.com = information about IMPAKT Communications and the literature and books published by IMPAKT.

- kyolic.com or estro-logic.com = information about the quality products manufactured and distributed by Wakunaga of America, manufacturers of Kyolic® brand aged garlic extract and Estro•Logic®, the menopause formula designed by Dr. Kathleen Fry and Claudia Wingo.

- questvitamins.com = information about the quality products manufactured and distributed by Quest Vitamins of Canada.

- womenshealth.com = the web site for Women's Health America, with information on natural estrogen replacement therapy.

- womensinternational.com = site for consulting pharmacists, compounding laboratory, and educational support.

RECOMMENDED
BOOKS AND PUBLICATIONS

1. Ahlgrimm M, Kells J: *The HRT Solution: Optimizing Your Hormone Potential.* Grand City Park, New York: Avery, 1999.

2. Anderson F: *Build Bone Health.* Green Bay: IMPAKT Communications, 1999.

3. Bender SD: *The Power of Perimenopause: A Woman's Guide to Physical and Emotional Health During the Transitional Decade.* New York: Three Rivers Press, 1998.

4. Crawford AM: *Herbal Remedies for Women.* Rocklin: Prima Publishing, 1997.

5. Crawford AM: *The Herbal Menopause Book.* Freedom: The Crossing Press, 1996.

6. Duke JA: *The Green Pharmacy.* Emmaus: Rodale Press, 1997.

7. Gaby A: *Preventing and Reversing Osteoporosis.* Rockdale: Prima Publishing, 1995.

8. Gladstar R: *Herbal Healing for Women.* New York: Simon & Schuster, 1993.

9. Grogan BC: *Soy Foods: Cooking for a Positive Menopause.* Summertown: Book Publishing Co., 1999.

10. Lark S: *The Estrogen Decision.* Berkeley: Self Help Books, 1995.

11. Laux M, Conrad C: *Natural Woman, Natural Menopause.* New York: HarperCollins, 1997.

12. McIntyre A: *The Complete Woman's Herbal*. New York: Henry Holt Publishing, 1994.

13. Northrup C: *Health Wisdom for Women Newsletter*. 7811 Montrose Rd., Potomac MD, 1-800-777-5005.

14. Northrup C: *Women's Bodies, Women's Wisdom*. New York: Bantam, 1995.

15. Tilford G: *From Earth to Herbalist*. Missoula: Mountain Tree Press Publishing Company, 1998.

16. Weed S: *Menopausal Years: The Wise Woman Way*. Woodstock: Ash Tree Publishing, 1992.

17. Wright J, Morganthaler J: *Natural Hormone Replacement*. Petaluma: Smart Publications, 1997.

18. Wright J, Gaby A: *The Patient's Book of Natural Healing*. Rockdale: Prima Publishing, 1999.

References

1. Ahlgrimm M, Kells J: *Restoring Balance: An Individualized Approach to Hormone Replacement Therapy*. Green Bay: IMPAKT Communications, 1998.

2. Albertazzi P, Pansini F, Bonaccorsi G, Zanotti L, Forini E, DeAloysio D: The effect of dietary soy supplementation on hot flashes. *Obstet Gynecol*, 1998.

3. Anderson F: *Build Bone Health: Prevent and Treat Osteoporosis*. Green Bay: IMPAKT Communications, 1999.

4. Anderson F, Gazella K: Evaluating osteoporosis treatment options. *Int J Integr Med*, Sep/Oct 1999.

5. Anderson JW, Johnstone BM, Cook-Newell ME: Meta-analysis of the effects of soy protein intake on serum lipids. *N Engl J Med*, Aug 1995.

6. Baird DD, Umbach DM, Lansdell L, Hughes CL, Setchell KD, Weinberg CR, Haney AF, Wilcox AJ, Mclachlan JA: Dietary intervention study to assess estrogenicity of dietary soy among postmenopausal women. *J Clin Endocrinol Metab*, May 1995.

7. Blumenthal M, *et al*: *German Commision E Monographs: Therapeutic Monographs of Medicinal Plants for Human Use*. Austin: American Botanical Council, 1998.

8. British Herbal Medicine Association: *British Herbal Pharmacopoeia*. BMHA, 1990.

9. Brown D: *Vitex agnus-castus* clinical monograph. *Quarterly Rev of Nat Med*, 1994.

10. Burghardt M: Exercise at menopause: a critical difference. *Medscape Women's Health*, 1999.

11. Cassidy A, Bingham S, Setchell, KDR: Biological effects of a diet of soy protein rich in isoflavones on the menstrual cycle of premenopausal women. *Am J Clin Nutr*, 1994.

12. Coope J: Hormonal and non-hormonal interventions for menopausal symptoms. *Maturitas*, 1996.

13. DeMarco C: *Take Charge of Your Body: Women's Health Advisor*. Winlaw: Well Women Press, Jul 1996.

14. Dennerstein L, Lehert P, Burger H, Dudley E: Mood and the menopausal transition. *J Nerv Ment Dis*, 1999.

15. Fleming T (ed): *Physicians Desk Reference*. Montvale: Medical Economics Company, 1998.

16. Gazella K: Menopause: natural alternatives to conventional estrogen. *Nature's Impact*, Oct/Nov 1997.

17. He ZP, Wang DZ, Shi LY, Wang ZQ: Treating amenorrhea in vital energy-deficient patients with Angelica sinensis-Astragalus membranaceus menstruation-regulating decoction. *J Tradit Chin Med*, Sep 1986.

18. Hong CY, Lo YC, Tan FC, Wei YH, Chen CF: Astragalus membranaceus and Polygonum multiflorum protect rat heart mitochondria against lipid peroxidation. *Am J Chin Med*, 1994.

19. Hobbs C: Black cohosh: a women's herb comes of age. *Herbs for Health*, Mar/Apr 1998.

20. Hunter A: *Cimicifuga racemosa*. National Herbalist Association of Australia, 1998.

21. Ingram D, Sanders K, Kolybaba M, Lopez D: Case-control study of phytoestrogens and breast cancer. *The Lancet*, Oct 1994.

22. Knight DC, Eden JA: A review of the clinical effects of phytoestrogens. *Obstet Gynecol*, May 1996.

23. Laux M, Conrad C: *Natural Woman, Natural Menopause*. New York: Harper Collins Publishers Inc., 1997.

24. Lieberman S: A review of the effectiveness of *Cimicifuga racemosa* (black cohosh) for the symptoms of menopause. *J Womens Health*, Jun 1998.

25. Liske E: Therapeutic efficacy and safety of *Cimicifuga racemosa* for gynecologic disorders. *Advances in Therapy*, 1998.

26. Lu LJW, Anderson KE, Grady JJ, Nagamani M: Effects of soya consumption for one month on steroid hormones in premenopausal women: implications for breast cancer risk reduction. *Cancer Epidemiol Biomarkers Prev*, 1996.

27. Mayo J, Mayo MA: Menopause imposters. *Int J Integr Med* 1(2):12-15, Mar/Apr 1999.

28. McTiernan A, *et al*: Prevalence and correlates of recreational physical activity in women aged 50-64 years. *Menopause*, 1998.

29. Milligan P: *Health Report Soy*. Green Bay: IMPAKT Communications, 2000.

30. Murkies AL, Lombard C, Strauss BJG, Wilcox G, Burger HG, Morton MS: Dietary flour supplementation decreases post-menopausal hot flashes: effect of soy and wheat. *Maturitas*, 1995.

31. Nagata C, Kabuto M, Kurisu Y, Shimizu H: Decreased serum estradiol concentration associated with high dietary intake of soy products in premenopausal Japanese women. *Nutr Cancer*, 1997.

32. Northrup C: *Women's Bodies, Women's Wisdom: Creating Physical and Emotional Health and Healing*. New York: Bantam Books, 1995.

33. Perry EK, Pickering AT, Wang WW, Houghton P, Perry NS: Medicinal plants and Alzheimer's disease: Integrating ethnobotanical and contemporary scientific evidence. *J Altern Complement Med*, 1998.

34. Potter SM: Soy protein and cardiovascular disease: the impact of bioactive components in soy. *Nutr Rev*, Aug 1998.

35. Potter SM, *et al*: Soy protein and isoflavones: their effects on blood lipids and bone density in postmenopausal women. *Am J Clin Nutr*, 1998.

36. Potter SM: Soy protein and serum lipids. *Curr Opin Lipidol*, Aug 1996.

37. Professional Perspectives: The future of integrative medicine. *Int J Integr Med*, Jan/Feb 2000.

38. Ringel M: Beyond hormones: other treatments for menopausal symptoms. *Patient Care*, Apr 1998.

39. Rozenberg S, Vandromme J, Ayata N, *et al*: Osteoporosis management. *Int J Fertil Women's Med*, 1999.

40. Schwingl PJ, Hulka BS, Harlow SD: Risk factors for menopausal hot flashes. *Obstet Gynecol*, 1994.

41. Skafar, Dxu R, Morales J, *et al*: Female sex hormones and cardiovascular disease in women. *J Clin Endocrinol Metab*, 1997.

42. Slaven L, Lee C: Mood and symptom reporting among middle-aged women: the relationship between menopausal status, hormone replacement therapy, and exercise participation. *Health Psychol*, 1997.

43. Stengler A, Stengler M: *Menopause Relief: Nature's Top Herbal Medicines and More*. Green Bay: IMPAKT Communications, 1998.

44. Stoll BA: Eating to beat breast cancer: potential role for soy supplements. *Ann Oncol*, Mar 1997.

45. Xia YX: The inhibitory effect of motherwort extract on pulsating myocardial cells in vitro. *J Tradit Chin Med*, Sep 1983.

Other booklets/books published by IMPAKT Communications:

BOOKLETS

- *Attention Deficit Disorder* by Jesse Lynn Hanley, M.D.
- *Build Strong Bones* by Angela Stengler, N.D., and Mark Stengler, N.D.
- *CoQ10* by Ray Sahelian, M.D.
- *Discover the Power of Aged Garlic Extract* by Rowan Hamilton, M.N.I.M.H., and Arnold Fox, M.D.
- *Drink Your Greens* by Mark Stengler, N.D.
- *Echinacea* by Mark Stengler, N.D.
- *Heart Disease* by Karolyn A. Gazella, featuring an interview with Kilmer McCully, M.D.
- *Kava* by Ray Sahelian, M.D.
- *Lipoic Acid* by Ray Sahelian, M.D.
- *Menopause Relief* by Angela Stengler, N.D., and Mark Stengler, N.D.
- *Natural Solutions for PMS* by Angela Stengler, N.D., and Mark Stengler, N.D.
- *Osteoarthritis* by Karolyn A. Gazella, featuring an interview with Jason Theodasakis, M.D.
- *Protecting the Prostate* by Jean-Yves Dionne, B.Sc., Phm., and Karolyn A. Gazella
- *Restoring Balance* by Marla Ahlgrimm, R.Ph., and John Kells
- *The Secret of St. John's Wort Revealed* by Jean-Yves Dionne, B.Sc., Phm., and Sherry Torkos, B.Sc., Phm.
- *Superior Healing Power of SAMe* by Sherry Torkos, B.Sc., Phm., and Karolyn A. Gazella

- *Vanish Varicose Veins* by Sherry Torkos, B.Sc., Phm.
- *Winning at Weight Loss* by Sherry Torkos, B.Sc., Phm., and Frances E. FitzGerald
- *Your Child's Health* by Angela Stengler N.D., and Mark Stengler, N.D.

BOOKS

- *Activate Your Immune System* by Leonid Ber, M.D., and Karolyn A. Gazella
- *Build Bone Health: Prevent and treat osteoporosis* by Freedolph Anderson, M.D.
- *Buyer Be Wise! The Consumer's Guide to Buying Quality Nutritional Supplements* by Karolyn A. Gazella
- *Devour Disease with Shark Liver Oil* by Peter T. Pugliese, M.D., with John Heinerman, Ph.D.

These booklets and books are available at your local health food store or by calling 800-477-2995 (U.S.) or 888-292-2229 (Canada).

www.impakt.com

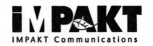

Health Information Specialists

www.impakt.com